AUTHORITY, OBSERVATION AND
EXPERIMENT IN MEDICINE

Authority, Observation and Experiment in Medicine

BY

W. W. C. TOPLEY

M.D., F.R.C.P., F.R.S.

*Professor of Bacteriology and Immunology
in the University of London*

LINACRE LECTURE 1940

CAMBRIDGE

AT THE UNIVERSITY PRESS

1940

CAMBRIDGE
UNIVERSITY PRESS

University Printing House, Cambridge CB2 8BS, United Kingdom

Published in the United States of America by Cambridge University Press, New York

Cambridge University Press is part of the University of Cambridge.

It furthers the University's mission by disseminating knowledge in the pursuit of
education, learning and research at the highest international levels of excellence.

www.cambridge.org
Information on this title: www.cambridge.org/9781107668713

© Cambridge University Press 1940

First published 1940
Re-issued 2014

A catalogue record for this publication is available from the British Library

ISBN 978-1-107-66871-3 Paperback

AUTHORITY, OBSERVATION
AND
EXPERIMENT IN MEDICINE

I T is a little over four hundred years since
Linacre founded his two lectureships, one
in his own University of Oxford and a
second at St John's College, Cambridge. An
invitation to fill this chair for one short hour
must, for old association's sake, be peculiarly
welcome to one whose undergraduate days
were spent at St John's. In my own case this
pleasure is increased by the fact that Dr Shore,
who directed my first steps in medical science
thirty-five years ago, is keeping his kindly eye
on my efforts to-day.

In his Rede Lecture, delivered in the last year
of peace, Sir Edward Mellanby sketched a
stimulating and provocative picture of recent
advances in medical science and of their social

and economic consequences. This evening, in the first year of war, I shall attempt to put forward some suggestions as to why those advances occurred, and how we can best ensure that they shall continue. Even in such an emergency as now confronts us there is, I think, something to be said for trying to define certain general principles, if only that we may better assess the significance of the host of crude, but instructive, administrative experiments that we are performing, or that are being performed on us, as war-time measures.

In this, as in all similar problems, we must learn from history if we are to learn at all, and we may well start with Linacre; for the significance of the things he did, or failed to do, lies in the fact that he lived, as we live to-day, at a turning point in the march of western civilisation. If we get a clear picture, even in outline, of what was happening to medicine in Linacre's day, and what has happened since, we shall be in a better position to grasp the meaning of what is happening now, and to determine how far, and in what direction, we can usefully interfere.

Two of my predecessors, Sir George Newman and the late Sir William Osler, devoted their lectures to a study of Linacre himself and of his influence on English medicine. It is with as much diffidence as regret, and with some feeling of ingratitude, that I admit my inability to accept the unqualified eulogies that they pronounced. As Browning's Grammarian, Linacre was one of the great pioneers of the new age of scholarship, and that, surely, is claim enough to immortality. As a physician, I cannot avoid the conclusion that the only reason he did no more harm than he did was because the times were too much for him. His was, I think, from the medical point of view, the high tragedy of the wrong thing supremely well done. His great achievement in medicine was the translation of much of Galen's Greek into admirable Latin. Galen had dominated medicine for thirteen hundred years, in life as a Greek physician in Rome, and after his death through his encyclopaedic writings, selections from which passed from one language to another as medical scholarship followed the fate of empires. The Ghost of Galen ruled over Arabian medicine, though such writers as Rhazes and Avicenna added many clinical observations and speculations of their own. It came back into Europe in the Latin texts and commentaries, derived from Arabian authors, which formed the basis of medical thought and teaching throughout the Middle Ages.

It was a corrupted Galen that Linacre found, and to him a corrupt text must have been a challenge that could not be refused. It was natural for him to believe that the resurrection of the Greek physician in his pristine purity would put medicine on the right road again. That great caution should be observed in dealing with the illustrious dead, and that their influence on those who came after them should be carefully pruned from year to year to make room for new growth, was not the kind of truth that would have appealed to the Linacre who is sketched for us in our very scanty records. But other men in Linacre's time were seeing the vision—it was as yet hardly more—to which he himself was blind. His Latin translations of Galen were published in the last years of his life, between 1517 and 1524. In 1527 a very different man was appointed Professor of Medicine in Basel. Paracelsus, as he called himself, or Theophrastus Bombastus von Hohenheim, to give him his baptismal name, was the son of a Swiss physician. He obtained his Doctor's degree at Ferrara, studying under Leonicenus who had, much earlier, been one of Linacre's Italian masters. Paracelsus had little of the scholar's temperament. He was among the last of the mediaeval alchemists, and may perhaps be reckoned among the forerunners of the modern chemists. He was a wanderer, who had picked up odd knowledge and odd friends in most parts of Europe, and his talk smacked of the tavern rather than of the study. But he knew better than Linacre what was wrong with medicine; and, if reports are true, he inaugurated his professorship at Basel by publicly burning the works of Galen and of Avicenna, and lecturing on medicine from his own experience, in his native tongue instead of in scholar's Latin. It is not often that the translating of books marks reaction, or the burning of books a new birth; but there can, I think, be little doubt that Linacre spent his labour in putting a brighter polish on the fetters that held medicine in thrall, or that the bonfire at Basel was as symbolic of freedom as the storming of the Bastille.

Of Linacre's other attempt at medical reform, the foundation of the Royal College of Physicians of London, I should naturally wish to speak with more enthusiasm; but, so far as its birth and babyhood are concerned, enthusiasm does not come easily to those who are thinking in terms of medical science. Its foundation marked an important professional victory. The Medical Act of 1511 had provided that no one should practise medicine in London, or within seven miles of its walls, except after examination and licence by the Bishop of London, or the Dean of St Paul's, with the aid of competent doctors of physic as assessors. When the College was founded in 1518, with Linacre as its first President, it assumed this privilege, and guarded it very jealously; but it is difficult to find evidence of any purposeful pursuit of new knowledge, or of any desire to break with professional dogma. In 1559, as Greenwood relates, an Oxford Doctor of Physic, John Geynes, dared to question the authority of Galen. He was required to bring to the notice of the College, within one month, all the passages in Galen's works that he deemed to be erroneous. Being a wise man he apologised instead.

Linacre the physician must, I think, be numbered among the authoritarians; and authority—the intellectual authority of books or men—is incompatible with science. The scientist can never regard his books as more than temporary codifications of current working hypotheses, and of the evidence on which they are based. All books, and all men, remain open to challenge, and there can be no plea of privilege.

If Linacre belonged to the night of medicine, which way was the dawn approaching? The break with authority which marked the rebirth, not of medicine alone, but of all effective human knowledge, was a thing that happened because the times were ripe for it. If one man's clarity of vision could have hastened events it might have happened three centuries before, when Roger Bacon anticipated the power of inductive and experimental science. Between his time and Linacre's the social and environmental factors that determine the responsiveness of men's minds to intellectual stimuli had undergone fundamental changes. The political and religious systems that had dominated Europe for centuries were breaking up, and new energies were being released on every side. But Linacre was no heir to Roger Bacon. That rôle belongs, by every sign and right, to a contemporary whom he may well have met in Florence.

Leonardo da Vinci was Linacre's senior by eight years, and died five years before him. His life is a lasting refutation of those who seek to place the artist and the scientist in different categories. As one item among his amazing range of activities he laid new foundations for anatomy, and for the observation of human structure in relation to function. To da Vinci anatomy was one among many interests. To Vesalius, who was born five years before da Vinci died, it was a life's work. If we had to select one man in the direct apostolic succession of medicine who marked the transit from the Middle Ages to the new world of human thought we should have to choose Vesalius, since he consciously, and in the teeth of opposition, cast off authority in favour of systematic observation. His *De Fabrica Humani Corporis*, published in 1543, put an end to many of the myths of Galenical anatomy, and cast more than a doubt on the working value of even the very best translations of the master's writings. Vesalius did not escape the common fate of medical reformers. Sylvius, who had taught him, attacked him with extreme violence, and, when confronted with some of Galen's more startling errors, gave it as his view that man's body must have changed, though not for the better.

Among the pupils of Vesalius was Fallopius, and among his pupils was Fabricius, and Fabricius taught a lively, dark-complexioned young

Englishman named William Harvey, who in 1598 had come from Cambridge to Padua to study medicine. With Harvey we take the decisive step, away from authority, through observation, to controlled experiment. The demonstration of the circulation of the blood, and the publication of *De Motu Cordis* in 1628, marks an advance even greater than that achieved by Vesalius, for it takes us past anatomy to physiology, and so to the beginnings of medical research in its fully effective form.

The outward careers of Linacre and Harvey were strangely alike. Each went to school at Canterbury, each studied medicine at Padua, each practised in London as Physician to the King. Linacre was the first President of the College of Physicians; Harvey was offered the Presidency, but refused it on account of age and infirmity. It is true that Linacre passed his undergraduate days at Oxford, Harvey at Cambridge, but the real difference between them was a difference in time. They belonged to different epochs. In Linacre's day the stream of knowledge that sprang from the replacement of authority by science was a trickle. That he failed to notice it is no matter for surprise. In Harvey's day many different streams were running for all to see. Copernicus had died half a century before Harvey was born. Galileo and Kepler were his contemporaries. William Gilbert recorded his experiments on terrestrial magnetism while Harvey was studying medicine in Padua. Boyle was thirty when Harvey died, and Newton a boy of fifteen. Science had begun a general, but ragged, advance.

If we follow the progress of medical science through the three centuries that separate Harvey's days from ours, I think that we shall at first be puzzled by its halting pace. In many aspects of clinical medicine there was, it is true, a slow but steady advance. Starting with Sydenham, whose life overlapped Harvey's, English clinicians began the laborious task of describing, and of differentiating from one another, the various diseases from which their patients suffered. In France, and in other countries, the same slow process of observation and classification was bringing order out of chaos. Towards the latter half of the eighteenth century the development of morbid anatomy, associated in this country with the name of John Hunter, began to add precision to the findings of the clinicians, and to afford a new and firmer basis for the differentiation of disease. Gradually there emerged a picture of diseases as separate clinical entities associated with certain diagnostic signs and symptoms and with characteristic changes in the patient's tissues. Nor was this advance in description and classification confined entirely to the field of medical practice as it affects the individual patient. Baillou in France and Sydenham in England gave a new impetus to epidemiology on the Hippocratic model, but they had few immediate followers. Not many physicians in the eighteenth century interested themselves in disease as it affects groups, instead of individuals, and of these only two added greatly to our knowledge—Pringle of the Army and Lind of the Navy, who described some of the diseases to which troops on land and crews at sea were particularly prone. The epidemiological descriptions of Sydenham had been pictorial, not quantitative. It was a contemporary of his, John Graunt, who brought statistics into medicine; but the seed that he sowed in the middle seventeenth century took nearly two hundred years to fructify.

Taken as a whole, this slow and fitful advance increased the accuracy of medical diagnosis, and made it more possible to forecast a patient's fate. But the causes of disease remained largely unknown, and the physician was almost as powerless as before to cure his patients or to prevent men falling sick. Why did effective knowledge come so slowly? I would suggest that two main factors were concerned.

To take the less important first. The practice of medicine was a highly organised profession long before Harvey's time, and advance in medical knowledge has been largely determined by the rules and conventions that have governed professional life. The medical profession has, throughout its history, shown two characteristic features. It has been highly individualistic, and it has been based on a system of varying financial rewards in the shape of fees from private patients. Medical competition has always existed. In Harvey's day it was as keen as in our own; and it would appear that its financial aspects were more dominant, at least in London. Among the rules at Harvey's own hospital of St Bartholomew's was one that forbade the apothecary to disclose the nature of the doctor's prescriptions. There was, it would seem, a brisk but illicit trade in the prescriptions, or "bills", of famous physicians. Harvey's own prescriptions do not seem to have been enhanced in value by his scientific eminence, since a contemporary remarks: "I knew several practitioners in this town who would not have given threepence for one of his bills." The average physician, who was no Harvey, but had a practice to build and to keep, could not be expected to give much time or thought to the advancement of knowledge, apart from increasing his own skill by the observation of such patients as consulted him at his hospital or in his private practice. Moreover, the same professional limitations tended to perpetuate that dependence on personal authority which renders scientific criticism ineffective, and allows opinion to pass as fact. Linacre's attempt to refurbish the Great God Galen had failed, and medicine had been liberated from enslavement to the dead, but a multitude of little Galens were left alive, and the fact that they spoke with a revealing discordancy did not greatly lessen the authority of any one of them within his own immediate circle. When two or more great men give two or more opinions, each backed solely by an appeal to an extensive, but undocumented, personal experience, knowledge can only halt until someone devises a method of discovering which signpost is pointing the right way.

As we noted above, it is particularly in regard to treatment that opinions tend to differ in the absence of effective knowledge. The great battle of the leeches, fought between Broussais and Louis in the Paris of the eighteen-thirties, affords one of the earliest examples of a planned attempt to confront therapeutic authority with a series of carefully recorded clinical observations. Broussais had a low opinion of the natural recuperative powers of the human body, and was a firm believer in active treatment. In all inflammatory diseases, including pneumonia, the right treatment in his view was to starve and to bleed. The best way to bleed was to leech, and to do it thoroughly, ten to fifty leeches a time. Leeches ran scarce in France. Under Broussais' stimulus the annual consumption rose in ten years from two million to forty-one million. It occurred to Louis, but apparently to nobody else, that it would be of interest to inquire whether those who were leeched recovered more often than those who were not. The results of his simple arithmetic gave no support to the leeches; and some, at least, of the sick were saved unnecessary discomfort. Louis applied his numerical method to other clinical problems, but he was before his time, and his command of statistical method was not sufficient to save him from falling into the traps set by small samples. Greenwood, who tells the story of his efforts, notes that Poisson was his contemporary, and invites us to guess what might have happened if Poisson's statistical genius had collaborated with Louis' desire to apply the test of numbers to clinical problems. Such a guess brings us directly to a consideration of the factor which was mainly responsible for the long lag in the growth of medical science.

Medicine is not a self-sufficing entity. It is, as we know it to-day, the application to the cure and prevention of disease of knowledge and of methods drawn from a wide variety of ancillary sciences—ancillary, be it noted, only in the sense that they have services to offer to medicine, not in the sense that their business is to be medicine's servants. Medicine, in fact, could never have advanced itself very effectively, or very far. It had to wait until other branches of science were ready to solve its fundamental problems and instruct it how to act. And so our inquiry as to why medicine halted so long after Vesalius and Harvey resolves itself into the problem as to why science in general progressed so slowly after the great days of Galileo, Gilbert, Newton and Boyle.

Perhaps it was partly because the eighteenth century was the century of reason, and of the encyclopaedists. The intelligentsia talked and wrote so much that they had little time or inclination for working in laboratories, even when they had laboratories in which to work. But that, I think, was not the real reason. Science was waiting for a new stimulus, and it was to come not from the disinterested inquirer after truth, but from the industrial revolution and the artisan. Professional medicine had never realised its need for more science. Industry, partly because it could define its problems in simpler and more concrete terms, partly because it was an empirical activity in which the actual results of any procedure were subjected to the coldest and most searching criticism, realised its needs more quickly and was able to make them felt. Black, the chemist, worked with Watt, the engineer, in Glasgow in the seventeen-sixties. When Farish started lecturing at Cambridge towards the close of the eighteenth century he gave a course on "arts and manufactures, more particularly such as relate to chemistry", and he had a laboratory equipped with a steam engine. Dalton carried out his experiments on marsh gas and matured his atomic theory in the ill-equipped laboratory provided for him by the Manchester Literary and Philosophical Society, which had earlier provided in its transient College of Arts and Sciences lectures on chemistry considered in its relation to arts and manufactures. The Royal Institution was founded by Count Rumford in 1799, under the auspices of the "Society for Bettering the Conditions of the Poor". It was specifically intended to facilitate the introduction of useful mechanical inventions and improvements, and to teach, by lectures and experiments, the application of science to the common purposes of life. The lectures became a feature of London society, but in its earlier days practical instruction was also given to artisans, and Davy and Faraday, who made the Institution famous, were both men of humble birth. The metamorphosis of science at the beginning of the nineteenth century was due to the evolution of a new class of salaried, whole-time scientists; men who, in addition to teaching what was already known, were expected to use the facilities provided for them in the advancement of knowledge within their special spheres. It became possible to make a career in science, and the doors were thrown open to ability from whatever class it came.

Before the middle of the nineteenth century physicists and chemists had provided an integrated body of experimental knowledge that made it possible to apply the methods they had devised to the study of biological problems, and so to pass from a description of living forms to the detailed study of function. It became possible, for the first time, to attack with some hope of success the problem of how a living organism works. Medicine, as a profession, was not ready to make use of such opportunities. Medical men might, and did, become scientists, but they were not scientists because they were medical men. Before the new knowledge could be applied effectively to the cure or prevention of disease, a new type of medical scientist had to develop, one who was prepared to forsake the practice of his profession with its attractive financial rewards, and to devote himself to the experimental study of physiology, and of those departures from physiological behaviour that underlie disease in all its forms.

It is characteristic of any branch of science entering on a phase of effective and rapid growth that it springs up almost simultaneously in many different places under the inspiration of many different men. If a pioneer has no immediate followers it is because his particular discovery has been made before its time. Germany and France were almost neck and neck in the race of the physiologists that started about the eighteen-forties. We, as is our habit, lagged a little behind. It was not until Michael Foster founded the Cambridge School of Physiology that we began to play a really serious part; but we may perhaps be forgiven for feeling that since then we have not done so badly.

If we had to choose one man as a pioneer of experimental mammalian physiology, most of us I fancy would point to Claude Bernard; but it was not Bernard alone who gave to Paris in the latter half of the nineteenth century its pre-eminence as a birthplace of new medical knowledge. While Bernard was showing us how the normal body works, Pasteur, a chemist, was giving experimental proof that the great range of departures from normal behaviour included in the category of infective disease result from the invasion of the body by micro-organisms. For four years, from 1873 to 1877, Bernard and Pasteur sat together in the French Academy of Medicine. It cannot often have happened that two such pioneers graced the same assembly at the same time.

We should not be adhering to the realist and objective canons that alone enable us to learn from history if we assumed that the physicians of Paris realised what was happening. "Physiology", remarked one of them, when Bernard was expounding his experimental findings, "can be of no practical use in medicine; it is but a *science de luxe*, which could well be dispensed with." Nor was the theory of the microbic origin of infective disease received with greater favour. More than five years later Duclaux, a gentle and courteous man, but wearied by his attempts to make his medical colleagues realise the significance of Pasteur's work, expressed his opinion of them in terms that lacked something of his usual kindliness. Lister, though himself a surgeon, did not find it much easier to convince the surgeons of London of the efficacy of the antiseptic method that he had based on Pasteur's earliest experiments.

And so we come almost to our own century, and to our own time. If we are to make any reference at all to the history of medicine during the last fifty years it can only be to note that more progress has been made than in all preceding ages put together. Our ability to treat disease, and to prevent it, has been transformed. It is true that there are still vast fields where we can do little more than our fathers did, because we have not yet gained the knowledge on which to act; but wherever we have been able to relate effects to their true causes, and to interfere intelligently instead of blindly with a morbid process, we have gained a control of an entirely different order from that available to earlier generations. There can be no difference of opinion as to how this has come about. No physician or surgeon would now refer to physiology, or pathology, or bacteriology, or biochemistry, as luxury sciences, irrelevant to practical medicine. No physiologist, or pathologist, or bacteriologist, or biochemist, with a knowledge of the facts, would deny that practising physicians and surgeons, drawing largely on knowledge gained by others, but applying and extending this knowledge within their own field, have achieved an advance that has revolutionised clinical medicine. The surgeon, having received the freedom of the internal tissues of the body from the bacteriologist, has exploited his new territory to the full, and with admirable results. The physician, utilising the methods of physiology in his study of the heart, or of the biochemist in dealing with metabolic disorders, or of the bacteriologist in solving the problems of infective disease, and adding the observations which his clinical experience enables him to make, has learned how to interfere effectively in a multitude of diseases that before defied his powers. Moreover, the action and reaction that always come into play when the methods of science are applied to practical ends have begun to produce their invariable effect. The clinician, applying the methods of the physiologist, has advanced physiology as well as clinical medicine. The academic scientist gains as much as he gives when he collaborates fruitfully with a clinical colleague.

There has, indeed, been so thorough a fusion between medical science and medical practice over a large part of the common field that I do not think that any one would find it an easy matter to define clinical medicine as it exists to-day, except in terms of a professional activity. Certainly the clinician of the middle nineteenth century has ceased to exist. No physician would now observe and treat his patients, in all their ills, guided only by his trained but unaided senses. Even when the methods actually employed demand little more than this, the knowledge on which they are based has usually been gained by a host of laboratory observations and experiments involving specialised scientific knowledge and elaborate technical equipment.

Turning to medical science as it is pursued in the laboratory, without immediate relation to events in the ward or in the field, the last fifty years, and particularly the years since the last great war, have seen an increasing integration between the biological and non-biological sciences in general, and between those sciences that are directly related to medicine and those that are not. The chemist and the physicist have come into medicine, and it is certain that they will stay with us, as colleagues on whose skill and knowledge we are becoming increasingly dependent.

All this is a cause for satisfaction; and, if any one suggests that medicine is doing reasonably well as it is, I think it would be very difficult to gainsay him. But it could certainly do better; and since change must come it would be foolish not to direct it if we can. What changes should we make, and what should we avoid, to gain more knowledge and to apply it more effectively?

So far as the basic medical sciences are concerned minor adjustments are required, rather than any fundamental change. There are still some barriers to be lowered, or surmounted, and some of us believe that laboratory workers must become more mobile, and that the ladders leading to the senior posts must be made less straight and narrow, if we are to escape from over-specialisation with its risks of sterility. A change that is clearly coming is the closer association of different research institutes, and different university departments, in organised attacks on particular medical problems. That means committees; and committees are dangerous things that need the most careful watching. I believe that a research committee can do one useful thing, and one only. It can find the workers best fitted, and most anxious, to attack a particular problem, bring them together, give them the facilities they need, and leave them to get on with the work. It can review progress from time to time, and make adjustments; but if it tries to do more, it will only do harm. The good committee is simply a mechanism for enabling individual research workers to function more effectively, and in closer touch with one another.

Where medical science merges with medical practice there is, I think, one good thing that better organisation can certainly do. Within my own life-time there has grown up a horrible monstrosity that I can only call shop-science, or in my own field of work, shop-pathology. Clinical workers, or epidemiologists, with no first-hand knowledge of the technical methods involved, or of the errors to which they are subject, order certain examinations to be made, and, having received the results, add them to the clinical data on which their working hypotheses, or diagnoses, are formed. If their clinical knowledge is less extensive than it might be, or the time they can spend in examining their patients is curtailed by press of practice, they can easily form the disastrous habit of relying on a collection of this second-hand information to give them all the data they require. It should be a rule permitting of very few exceptions that, if a clinical or epidemiological problem demands technical methods that the clinician or epidemiologist cannot himself apply, there should be personal contact between all those concerned in arriving at a solution. I do not mean, of course, that there must be personal consultation over every specimen examined, or over every case. But all those concerned must be in constant personal touch, and know enough of one another's methods to talk a common language. They must work as members of a team, not as buyers and sellers of information. In our large teaching hospitals this particular problem has been solved; but in many smaller hospitals, in general practice, and in the work of many public health authorities, its solution must await the provision of laboratory services on a greatly extended scale, and with a far higher degree of co-ordination.

No one, I think, will deny that it is from the laboratory that the great medical discoveries will come in the future as they have come in the past. There is no way of gaining new knowledge so effective as controlled experiment, and no substitute for it. When we find a cure for cancer, or tuberculosis, as effective as insulin in diabetes, the arsenicals in syphilis, or the sulphanilamide compounds in certain bacterial infections, it will be because someone has done something in a laboratory. Whatever else we do, we must maintain and increase the continuous pressure of new facts, and new theories, which the laboratory worker exerts on medical science.

If any of us were asked, not what kind of medical research it is most important to maintain, but what field of medical research is most in need of development, I think we should probably agree that it is on the applied side that there is most room for improvement in our present ways of doing things.

Some of you may have felt that I have laid needless stress on the lack of sympathy, sometimes amounting to antagonism, which characterised the relations between medical practice and medical science until quite recent times. To ignore it would have been to ignore an essential factor in the problem which faces us to-day, though not in the form in which it faced our fathers. There are, I think, two main influences that have hindered, and to some extent still hinder, the full and close co-operation of all those engaged in studying, preventing, or curing human disease. One, to use a current catchword, is ideological, the other is severely practical.

Among the many phrases that have done all the harm that words can do, I doubt if any has been more mischievous than that dreadful double label—the science and art of medicine. The essence of science is method; and, if art means craft, there can be no mutually exclusive definition of the methods by which the scientist and the craftsman pursue their ends. There is only one way of increasing effective knowledge: the method of working hypothesis, prediction and trial. On the basis of a series of observations we evolve a hypothesis. On the basis of this hypothesis we predict that, under specified conditions, we shall be able to observe a specified event. We attempt to secure the conditions and see whether our prediction comes true. If it does, our hypothesis becomes more

«[35]»

probable. If it does not we may discard our hypothesis, or alter it, or doubt whether we have really secured the specified conditions, or whether our final observation has been correctly made, and we may start again. What we must never do is to leave our hypothesis untested, or neglect the results of our tests without showing why they failed. This essential process underlies the work of the clinical observer just as it underlies that of his colleague in the laboratory. The physician, on the basis of a series of observations made on a sick person, forms a working hypothesis which he labels a diagnosis. By deduction from his hypothesis he makes a prediction which he labels a prognosis: the patient will recover, wholly or partially, or he will die, or he will respond to such and such treatment in such and such a way. The physician becomes a sound scientist, and surely a sound clinician, if, and only if, he completes the process by noting whether his prediction comes true. This means a careful follow-up of his patients when they live, or, if they die, a personal attendance at a post-mortem if this can be obtained. Looking back on some of my own teachers, my conviction is strengthened that, given equal innate capacities, clinicians become great, or fail to do so, according as they obey or disregard this first principle of scientific empiricism.

Sometimes the term artist is used to denote a man who does a particular thing supremely well, in virtue of natural endowments raised to their highest effectiveness by training and experience. By some the scientist is regarded as a man who, working by well-tried rules of logic and experiment, has made himself independent of artistry or intuition. This is entirely false. The really great scientist is always a great artist. He observes things to which lesser men are blind, sees implications that other men ignore, forms hypotheses that look like guesses but have an uncanny way of proving true, and, when he goes wrong, learns more from his mistakes than others do from their successes. By some the artist is regarded as a man who owes little or nothing to working hypotheses or experimental tests. This is an even more dangerous fallacy. A worker in a laboratory who, when he performs an illuminating experiment, fails to realise that he is proving himself an artist, loses only a tickle to his personal vanity. A physician who, regarding himself as an artist, fails to realise that he is performing a series of peculiarly difficult experiments, is not likely to add greatly to his own knowledge or that of others.

Science has tried and condemned authority, and in its grosser forms authority is dead. Where it still lives in the field of medicine it might, I think, be defined as the didactic assertion of inadequately tested working hypotheses, accompanied by an unwillingness to meet the challenge of a critic by performing a more adequate series of tests.

These tests must all be of the same essential kind; predictions that, under such-and-such conditions, so-and-so will happen, and a demonstration that, in fact, it does. Sometimes the thing that happens is an event in which the observer takes no active part, sometimes it is a result that he produces by a calculated interference with the natural course of events. The first kind of test we often call an observation, the second an experiment. It is a useful distinction, but I think it is a dangerous one.

Darwin, you will remember, laid great stress on the significance of variation under domestication in relation to the origin of species by natural selection. He emphasised the tendency of highly modified varieties to revert to the ancestral type on crossing. He records that he crossed white fantail pigeons with black barbs, and a barb with a spot. On crossing a fantail-barb mongrel with a barb-spot mongrel he obtained a typical blue rock pigeon, with the double black bar on its wings and barred tail feathers. Just as he believed the rock pigeon to be the ancestor of all our domestic races, Darwin concluded, from a series of observations, that the remote common ancestor of our various breeds of horses had zebra-like stripes. Predicting that, if this were so, some breeds of horses would show the facial stripe of the zebra, as well as stripes on the body and legs, he asked Colonel Poole whether the Kattywar breed of horses, known to show frequent stripings, was ever striped on the face, and received an affirmative answer. Was Darwin performing an experiment when he crossed his barbs, spots and fantails, but not when he questioned Colonel Poole? It may be so; but I should myself prefer to regard the interrogation of the Colonel as an experiment of a crude but effective kind, if only to emphasise the unity of the scientific method of prediction and test.

A great part of clinical medicine, and of epidemiology, must still be observation. Nature makes the experiments, and we watch and understand them if we can. No one will deny that we should always aim at planned intervention and closer control. Here, as elsewhere, technique—the way we make our observations and check them—is half the battle; but to force experiment and observation into sharply separated categories is almost as dangerous a heresy as the science and art antithesis. It tends to make the clinician in the ward, the epidemiologist in the field, and the laboratory worker at his bench, think of themselves as doing different things, and bound by different rules. Actually they are all making experiments, some good, some bad. It is more difficult to make a good experiment in the ward than in the laboratory, because conditions are more difficult to control; but there is no other way of gaining knowledge. If we could kill the last remnants of authoritarianism, abolish the false distinction between the medical scientist and the medical artist, and gain general acceptance for the view that controlled observation in the ward or in the field is an essential part of medical science, shading through almost imperceptible stages of increasing intervention into the fully developed experimental technique of the laboratory, we should, I am sure, have gone a long way to secure the intellectual sympathy and understanding that is the essential basis of fruitful common effort.

So much for ideological influences. Now for the severely practical. What I have been saying would make strange hearing to the zoologist or botanist. It would never occur to him that field studies were an art, experiments at the bench a science; that all the fundamental rules were changed as one went in or out of the laboratory door. There is, I think, no doubt that the clash which, even more than the clash of mistaken ideologies, underlies our relative failure to exploit the potentialities of clinical science is the professional clash between medical practice and clinical research. It would be utterly unjust to charge consulting physicians or surgeons, or general practitioners, with any negligence in not devoting more of their time to the advancement of clinical knowledge. They are not paid to advance knowledge. They are paid to look after their patients, and the more patients they look after the more they are paid. In spite of the claims of private practice, the consultants attached to our great teaching hospitals devote much of their time to teaching; and in the course of their hospital or private practice many of them make, and put on record, observations of the greatest value. It is they, and their predecessors, who have raised practical medicine and surgery to the high level of the present day. It is true that most consultants have not the time for the detailed and prolonged study of their patients, for the discussions with their laboratory colleagues, or for the extensive reading and thinking, which are essential for the full development of clinical research; but we cannot expect, and certainly shall not get, active and sustained research as a casual by-product of a busy professional life.

We noted, when we were considering the sudden acceleration in the growth of science at the beginning of the nineteenth century, that it was due, in the main, to the emergence of a new class of salaried professional scientists, paid to devote their whole time to teaching and research. We need have no doubts that the same stimulus, applied on an adequate scale to the clinical science of to-day, would produce the same results. The whole-time salaried clinical teacher and investigator has, indeed, already proved his worth. It is an equally safe prophecy that no other stimulus will have any significant effect.

I know that, in suggesting changes in the

organisation of clinical practice, I am trespassing well beyond my proper sphere; but I take courage from the fact that our Regius Professor of Physic has recently put on record conclusions which, so far as I can judge, differ in no essentials from my own.

I would add one thing more. The advancement of clinical science is usually discussed in terms of the teaching hospital. It is sometimes discussed as though the problems of disease were confined within hospital walls. In fact, many of the problems that most need solving can only be attacked by observing people in their own homes, or at their work, and over long periods of time. Any organisation that fails to provide the general practitioner with increased opportunities for adding to our knowledge of disease will leave untouched one of the major deficiencies of the existing system. Perhaps the various schemes of regionalised medical services that are now being explored will afford an opportunity for doing something along these lines.

To what extent hospital medical practice

could, with advantage, be put on a whole-time salaried basis is a problem on which there will certainly be differences of opinion. Whatever happens, it is likely that any possible transition from a fee-earning to a salaried profession will be a slow one; and that, perhaps, is a good thing. Unless we move cautiously, regarding each new step as an experiment, and testing it by its results, we may find ourselves caught in a bureaucratic net that will be little to our liking.

Whatever system we adopt, it must be kind to rebels, and there must be no good-conduct prizes. It is, of course, not true that whole-time salaries are incompatible with initiative, or with freedom to criticise. I have not observed that my colleagues among University Professors and Lecturers have lost the power of criticising one another, or the administrative systems under which they work. I hope they never will. Nor have I observed that meekness gets many marks when senior appointments are being made. It should be possible, within reason, to devise an administrative machine that will deliver the conditions of work required, provided that we do not ask it to turn out incompatible products. We have, I think, some models that are worth copying, or adapting. We have others that show us, with the utmost clarity, what to avoid.

Whatever plans we make will, in the end, depend on education. If we do not train our students to think for themselves—perhaps it would be fairer to say, if we do not allow them to think for themselves—no opportunities that we provide in later life will be of much avail. With an overloaded curriculum it is no easy thing to avoid didactic teaching. It takes much longer to allow a student to observe things for himself than to tell him what he ought to find. Some students still make debatable assertions at their final examinations on the sole ground, which they have come to regard as entirely adequate, that Mr Blank has told them so. I am not sure that the Ghost of Galen has yet been wholly exorcised from our medical schools.

9 781107 668713